The LITTLE PROTEIN COOKBOOK

THE LITTLE PROTEIN COOKBOOK

Copyright © Octopus Publishing Group Limited, 2025

All rights reserved.

Text by Benjamin Benton

No part of this book may be reproduced by any means, nor transmitted, nor translated into a machine language, without the written permission of the publishers.

Condition of Sale
This book is sold subject to the condition that it shall not, by way of trade or otherwise, be lent, resold, hired out or otherwise circulated in any form of binding or cover other than that in which it is published and without a similar condition including this condition being imposed on the subsequent purchaser.

An Hachette UK Company
www.hachette.co.uk

Vie Books, an imprint of Summersdale Publishers
Part of Octopus Publishing Group Limited
Carmelite House
50 Victoria Embankment
LONDON
EC4Y 0DZ
UK

This FSC® label means that materials used for the product have been responsibly sourced

www.summersdale.com

The authorized representative in the EEA is Hachette Ireland, 8 Castlecourt Centre, Dublin 15, D15 XTP3, Ireland (email: info@hbgi.ie)

Printed and bound in Poland

ISBN: 978-1-83799-480-9

> Substantial discounts on bulk quantities of Summersdale books are available to corporations, professional associations and other organizations. For details contact general enquiries: telephone: +44 (0) 1243 771107 or email: enquiries@summersdale.com.

The LITTLE PROTEIN COOKBOOK

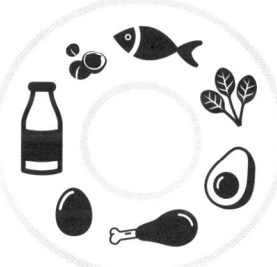

Taylor Spencer

DISCLAIMER

Neither the author nor the publisher can be held responsible for any injury, loss or claim – be it health, financial or otherwise – arising out of the use, or misuse, of the suggestions made herein. Always consult your doctor before trying any new diet if you have a medical or health condition, or are worried about any of the side effects. This book is not intended as a substitute for the medical advice of a doctor or physician.

Contents

INTRODUCTION..................................7

THE BASICS......................................8

RECIPES

    BREAKFAST..............................26
    LUNCH......................................42
    DINNER....................................64
    DESSERT..................................90
    SNACKS..................................102

MEAL PLANNERS..........................114

CONCLUSION................................122

INTRODUCTION

Welcome to *The Little Protein Cookbook*. This book is a pocket-sized introduction to a high-protein diet. A high-protein diet involves eating more protein (this can be meat, but just as easily plant protein), which often leads to a reduction in your fat and carbohydrate intake.

Following this diet can support weight loss, but its other benefits relate more to general health, such as suppressing appetite hormones (leaving you fuller for longer), stabilizing blood sugar levels, improving your overall energy and, of course, supporting growth and strength.

Whether the idea of a high-protein diet is new to you or you follow a similar regime already, this book will give you an overview of the diet and the importance of protein, followed by recipes for breakfast, lunch, dinner, dessert and even snacks, plus three seven-day meal planners to help you work a high-protein diet into your day-to-day.

THE BASICS

This chapter covers the basics of a high-protein diet. It looks at the benefits of the diet, what the diet might consist of and how to get started. It will also touch on the protein content of foods like meat, fish, fruit, vegetables, oats, seeds and legumes. It also covers supplements, which are another way to add protein to your diet, and how to track or monitor your protein. Finally, it offers a very simple list of dos and don'ts that will help you on your high-protein journey.

WHAT IS A HIGH-PROTEIN DIET?

A high-protein diet is one in which 20 per cent of your daily intake of calories consists of protein. Protein comes in many forms and can be derived from meat, fish, dairy, beans, pulses, nuts, seeds, eggs and certain grains such as quinoa. By focusing more of your diet on these high-protein foods, you will naturally lean away from carbs, especially refined carbs that tend to be higher in sugar – such as pasta, bread and other baked goods. A good rule of thumb is to aim to consume 15–30 g of protein per meal, four to five times a day. Your body can only absorb 30 g of protein at any one time, so massively exceeding this will just see the protein pass straight through your body.

While a high-protein diet involves increasing the amount of protein you eat, in reality it is often achieved by replacing carbohydrates with protein. The degree to which you reduce or remove carbohydrates from your meals to achieve a high-protein intake is up to you. Notable high-protein diets such as the Atkins and Duke diets espouse removing almost all carbohydrates from your diet, whereas the paleo and keto diets remove most carbohydrates while focusing on eating protein along with good unsaturated fats, such as those found in oily fish, eggs and avocados.

It is important to note that while high-protein diets can help reduce hunger, boost the rate at which we burn calories, and increase muscle mass, completely removing any food group, such as carbohydrates, from your diet should only ever be done under medical supervision as it can negatively alter your gut microbiota, which can have a detrimental effect on the gut and your overall health.

WHY IS PROTEIN IMPORTANT?

Every cell in our bodies needs protein. Proteins are made up of building blocks called amino acids, and an adequate amount of protein intake is important for keeping our muscles, bones and tissues healthy. Protein, crucially, is one of the major energy-giving nutrients we consume, which might seem at odds with the common notion that carbohydrate intake is the main way to boost our energy.

Protein plays many vital roles in maintaining our health, including aiding muscle strength, helping our bodies heal, making new cells and repairing old ones. Protein also plays a vital role in creating the hormones and enzymes that carry out key functions for us day in, day out.

There are thousands of different proteins in our body and many sources of protein that we can consume. Each type of protein contains its own mix of amino acids, with each amino acid bringing a crucial characteristic to the party. As with anything to do with our diet, variety really is key. So, eating a wide range of proteins from various sources will ensure you have a healthy, balanced diet.

WHAT ARE THE BENEFITS OF A HIGH-PROTEIN DIET?

While the three main macronutrients in our diets – carbohydrates, fat and protein – all offer different benefits, studies show that protein fills us up for longer. In terms of the science, protein reduces the hunger hormone ghrelin and increases peptide YY, the hormone that makes you feel full.

Additionally, one of protein's core skills – and perhaps its most well-known trait – is that it forms the building blocks of our muscle mass. Eating a high-protein diet combined with physical activity, such as strength training, can lead to an impressive increase in your muscle mass. Similarly, keeping your protein intake high while losing weight will ensure you don't lose muscle mass as the weight drops off.

Beyond these two major benefits, eating a high-protein diet can reduce cravings, boost your metabolism and burn fat, lower your blood pressure, and help your body repair itself.

HOW MUCH PROTEIN IS TOO MUCH?

The amount of protein we each need depends on factors such as our age, weight and physical make-up and how active we are. A healthy, balanced diet should already be providing you with all the protein you need. However, there are clear benefits to eating more protein than we strictly need.

But can we have too much protein? It used to be that high-protein diets prompted fears around kidney, heart and bone health as a result of increased protein consumption. Largely, though, these fears have been disproved by science. Studies have found no link between high-protein diets and heart disease, and the same can be said for bone health too. High-protein diets do increase the workload for the kidneys, yet research shows that anyone with normal kidney function won't be negatively affected. If you have kidney disease, however, you should not adopt a high-protein diet as it can increase the rate at which kidney function declines.

The recommended daily intake for protein consumption for adults is 0.8 g per kilo of body weight in the US and 0.75 g per kilo of body weight in the UK.

MEAT OR PLANT PROTEIN?

Proteins are made up of amino acids, and while your body can make some nonessential amino acids, it cannot produce all the essential amino acids you need. This means you need to consume certain foods to get them. While each protein has a slightly different make-up, you can get all the amino acids you need from either plants or meat.

The main differentiating factor is what else is included in those foods besides the proteins. High-protein diets are often associated with muscle gain. This is because animal proteins can be more effective at building muscle mass as they deliver complete amino acids that help stimulate muscle growth. But while meat will have all the amino acids you need, it is more likely to contain unhealthy fats and no fibre.

Plant-based proteins can deliver the same amino acids, but they may require you to eat more of them to deliver the same effect. This can involve taking in more carbohydrates.

Plant-based proteins are also often wrapped in fibre that is harder for our bodies to break down.

Eating a wide variety of foods – and especially whole, unprocessed foods – seems to achieve the healthiest balance while meeting all our protein needs. Studies conclusively show that following a vegetarian or vegan diet does not mean you can't get the proteins you need, nor does it mean having to forgo a high-protein diet. Eat protein from as many sources as you can, and you'll be setting yourself up just fine.

WHAT ARE PROTEIN SUPPLEMENTS?

Protein supplements often come in the form of a powder that you can use to make shakes or add to recipes; protein bars are also popular. More often than not the supplements are made from whey or plant proteins, but they can also be derived from meat sources.

At first glance, protein supplements might seem like an easy way to add protein to your diet. They're certainly convenient, but beware the cost. A quick analysis of the price per kilogram of protein powder versus other whole-food proteins shows that protein supplements can easily be from two to 20 times more expensive per gram of protein.

Supplements are popular among those pursuing either weight management or muscle growth, as the hunger-suppressing nature of protein combined with its muscle-building qualities leads to results. And adding a supplement to your diet can be much easier than having to suddenly become your own personal chef and bulk-meal prepper. However, there are other downsides, such as the addition of some contaminants and sugars or sweeteners, as well as the risk of excessive protein intake. Eating whole foods will always be a more sustainable and healthy way to adopt a high-protein diet.

Protein supplements can be a good way to add a protein boost to meals, but they should only ever be a supplement to a good diet already packed with whole-food proteins.

WHEN SHOULD I EAT PROTEIN?

Consuming protein first thing in the morning is a great way to get an energy boost and set yourself up for the day. While some people may start the day with huge quantities of eggs, milk, yoghurt and protein shakes to boost their breakfast routine, this isn't necessary. Starting the day with a high-protein breakfast should leave you feeling fuller and less hungry as you go through the morning, but spreading your protein intake throughout the day can be the best way to approach a high-protein diet as your body can only absorb 30 g of protein at any one time, so consuming more than this will have no additional impact.

Many high-protein diets suggest consuming your protein in four to five portions throughout the day. For most of us this would look like breakfast, lunch and dinner, plus two protein-rich snacks, shakes, or even desserts, to arrive at our optimum protein intake. For those of us wanting to adopt a high-protein diet as part of a physically active lifestyle or alongside weight training, protein should be consumed within two hours of being active or working out to aid recovery and promote the growth of muscle cells.

HOW CAN I TRACK MY PROTEIN INTAKE?

There are a variety of websites and apps that can help you track your daily protein intake. These require you to enter detailed information about what you have eaten. The tracker will then tell you your "macros" or the make-up of the macronutrients you have consumed, protein included.

Perhaps the most common way to track your protein intake is to make a note of the protein content of the meals, snacks and shakes that you regularly consume. Those who eat a high-protein diet over a long period of time will have a selection of go-to foods and meals that they know will each deliver 15–30 g of protein. By combining these throughout the day, they can be confident that they're working towards their recommended daily intake.

You will start to notice that eating a banana, a serving of Greek yoghurt and a hard-boiled egg will deliver you approximately 19 g of protein for breakfast; a chicken breast with a portion of rice and vegetables amounts to around 25 g of protein; and a bean and brown rice burrito with cheese and avocado delivers about 28 g of protein.

It is worth reiterating that protein should accompany fruits, vegetables and whole grains; it should not be the entire meal. If you want to increase your protein intake without tracking it specifically, always start by adding more beans, lentils, soya or seafood rather than processed supplements.

ARE THERE ANY INSTANT PROTEIN WINS?

Dairy tends to be the quickest shortcut to a protein boost. Adding milk to smoothies or eating cheese as a snack or cottage cheese or cream cheese as a dip with fruit and veg are all super-easy protein wins. If you can't drink cows' milk, seek out a soya alternative for a protein boost as oat, rice and almond milks don't have nearly the protein content of cows' or soya milk.

Another easy win is to substitute your simple carbs, such as rice and pasta, for whole grains high in protein, such as quinoa. Not only is quinoa a high-protein hero, it also has more fibre and is more nutritious than its counterparts.

Having snacks like biltong or jerky, hard-boiled eggs, or nuts is a great way to ensure you have an instant protein win when you're out and about. In terms of nuts, leaning towards unsalted peanuts, almonds, pistachios, Brazil nuts, walnuts and cashews will give you the best high-protein boost for your money.

Finally, smoothies are a great way to get an almost instant protein boost. As mentioned previously, adding milk or yoghurt is a winner, as are seeds such as chia and hemp, which are both protein powerhouses.

HOW MUCH PROTEIN IS IN STAPLE FOOD ITEMS?

FOOD ITEM	PORTION SIZE	PROTEIN CONTENT
Chicken breast	120 g	33 g protein
Beef mince	140 g	28 g protein
Lamb chops	140 g	40 g protein
Tofu	120 g	28 g protein
Salmon	100 g	23 g protein
Tinned tuna	1 x 110-g can (drained)	28 g protein
Baked beans	1 x 400-g can	18.5 g protein
Green lentils	120 g	12 g protein
Chickpeas	120 g	10 g protein
Spinach	100 g	4 g protein
Cheddar	80 g	20 g protein
Mozzarella	50 g	11 g protein

FOOD ITEM	PORTION SIZE	PROTEIN CONTENT
Cows' milk	½ pint	10 g protein
Soya milk	½ pint	9 g protein
Yoghurt	125 g	7 g protein
Boiled eggs	2 medium eggs	14 g protein
Pumpkin seeds	30 g	10 g protein
Unsalted roasted peanuts	50 g	12 g protein
Peanut butter	25 g	6 g protein

A HIGH-PROTEIN DIET: DOs

- **Include protein in every meal:** Planning meals around a protein – such as lean meat, beans or eggs – and filling the rest of the plate with vegetables is a healthy and sustainable way to eat more protein while also getting a balance of nutrients in your diet.

- **Reduce your reliance on processed carbs:** Instead of instinctively reaching for white rice, pasta and bread to bulk out a meal, expand your dry stores to include whole grains high in protein, like quinoa. You could also replace pasta with strips of courgette or carrot, and substitute rice for crumbled cauliflower, barley or bulgur wheat.

- **Snack on protein:** Reaching for nuts, cheese and dips such as hummus is much better for sating your appetite when hunger strikes between meals.

- **Start your day with protein:** Focus on high-protein breakfast foods like eggs and smoothies made with protein powder, such as whey, pea protein or collagen.

A HIGH-PROTEIN DIET: DON'Ts

- **Assume all proteins are the same:** Pork has a high concentration of saturated fats, beef has plenty of iron on top of the saturated fats, and sausages and salami often have added nitrates and salt. Lean sources of protein are best, such as chicken, salmon, eggs, kefir, yoghurt, beans and legumes.

- **Exclusively eat protein:** Protein can work wonders, but not by itself. If you eat only protein, your body is deprived of other nutrients that it needs to function healthily. For instance, your body needs carbohydrates to stay healthy because they are the primary source of fibre and antioxidants that are crucial to help reduce the risk of diseases such as type 2 diabetes, colon cancer and obesity. Carbs also provide energy, so they are essential if you are very active.

- **Consume all your daily protein in one meal:** Consuming a lot of protein in one sitting can harm your kidneys by forcing them to work harder than usual. Instead, divide your proteins across your meals throughout the day.

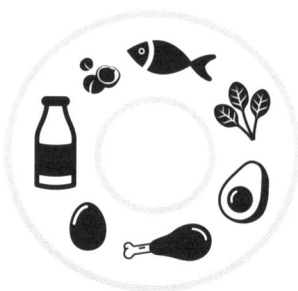

BREAKFAST

It stands to reason that getting plenty of protein in your first meal of the day is a surefire way to achieve a high-protein diet, but there are other benefits too.

Including plenty of protein in your breakfast will help you feel fuller and more satisfied as you go through the morning.

You may well be getting plenty of protein in your breakfast anyway, as lots of wholemeal breads and full-fibre cereals contain protein. If you're enjoying milk, yoghurt, eggs, fish or meat already as part of your breakfast, these are all great for a morning protein boost.

In this chapter we will build on the breakfast protein classics and give you some fun and delicious ideas for high-protein breakfasts to add to your repertoire.

Cowboy beans and poached eggs

Think of these cowboy beans as a slightly pimped-up version of baked beans. Make a big batch, doubling or tripling the amounts here, so that you have them ready in the fridge.

Serves 2

Contains 29 g of protein per serving

INGREDIENTS

100 g lardons
1 garlic clove, sliced
1 tsp dried chilli flakes
1 x 400-g can butter beans, drained
100 g passata
2 large tomatoes, chopped
½ tsp salt
1 tbsp vinegar
4 eggs

METHOD

Heat a heavy-bottomed pan over a medium heat and fry the lardons until golden brown. Add the garlic and chilli flakes and allow to cook for a minute or two. Next, add the drained butter beans, passata, chopped tomatoes and ¼ tsp salt and reduce to a simmer for 1 hour.

Once the sauce has reduced and thickened, bring a large pan of water to the boil over a medium heat and add the vinegar. Swirl the simmering water with a wooden spoon and crack in the eggs one by one. Cook for 3 minutes before removing with a slotted spoon and draining on a kitchen towel. Season the eggs with the remaining salt and serve two per person with a nice spoonful of the cowboy beans.

Mexican divorced eggs

Nothing says high-protein breakfast like eggs, and in this classic Mexican staple they are supercharged with two salsas, so you're pumped for the day ahead.

Serves 2

Contains 17 g of protein per serving

INGREDIENTS
FOR THE SPICY TOMATO SALSA:

1 tbsp olive oil
½ red onion, chopped
½ garlic clove, minced
1 red chilli, chopped
½ tsp ground allspice
400 g ripe tomatoes, chopped
¼ tsp salt

FOR THE GREEN APPLE SALSA:

1 Granny Smith apple, chopped
½ cucumber, chopped
1 handful of coriander leaves, chopped
2 spring onions, chopped

1 green chilli, chopped   **¼ tsp salt**
2 limes, juiced

YOU WILL ALSO NEED:

olive oil
4 eggs

METHOD

To make the tomato salsa, heat the oil in a heavy-bottomed pan and fry the onion and garlic over a medium heat until soft. Add the chilli and allspice and continue to cook for a few minutes before adding the tomatoes. Leave to cook over a low heat for a few minutes while you combine all the ingredients for the green salsa in a small bowl and season to taste. Finally, add a splash of oil to a frying pan over a high heat to make crispy eggs. Crack in the eggs and season each yolk with a little salt. As the eggs start to bubble and crisp, spoon over the excess oil in the pan to cook them evenly. As soon as all the white is cooked, transfer the eggs to two plates; spoon the tomato salsa over one half of the eggs and the green salsa over the other half.

Breakfast bread

A protein-packed breakfast bread that is easy to throw together, freezes well and is a delicious start to the day.

10 servings

Contains 16 g of protein per serving

INGREDIENTS

5 large overripe bananas
200 g ground almonds
125 g buckwheat flour
2 scoops protein powder
60 g maple syrup
60 g chia seeds
60 g sunflower seeds
1 tbsp peanut butter
1 tbsp molasses
2 eggs

METHOD

Preheat the oven to 170°C and line a loaf tin with baking parchment. Start by mashing the bananas in a large mixing bowl. Add the rest of the ingredients one by one, thoroughly mixing each time. Transfer the batter to the lined loaf tin and place in the oven for 60-75 minutes, or until a skewer inserted into the centre of the bread comes out clean. Cool on a wire rack. Serve slices of the bread toasted with butter, or indeed any topping of your choice. Mashed banana and almond butter work particularly well.

Mexican chia and chocolate breakfast shake

Packed with protein from the chia, this is a sharp and fruity shake that has a little kick from the cacao.

Serves 2

Contains 35 g of protein per serving

INGREDIENTS

- 1 handful of spinach
- 1 banana, chopped
- 200 g watermelon, chopped
- 200 g strawberries, hulled
- 1 tbsp chia seeds
- 1 tbsp cacao powder
- 2 scoops protein powder
- 1 lime, juiced
- 240 ml whole milk

METHOD

Simply add everything to your blender and blitz ferociously until you have a nice smooth shake.

Very berry breakfast bowl

Sometimes you just need a lift from a big pink bowl of comforting goodness – and that is exactly what this is.

Serves 2

Contains 34 g of protein per serving

INGREDIENTS

- 1 banana, chopped
- 2 cooked beetroots, chopped
- 200 g strawberries, hulled
- 2 tbsp rye oats
- 2 tbsp Greek yoghurt
- 2 scoops protein powder
- 200 ml whole milk
- 200 g berries (fresh or frozen), to top
- 50 g pecans, chopped, to top

METHOD

Add all the ingredients to a blender and blitz to a bright, smooth breakfast yoghurt. Transfer into two bowls, and top with berries of your choice and some chopped pecans.

Shakshuka and baked eggs

Having a few egg-based breakfasts is a smart move in the pursuit of a high-protein and high-deliciousness diet, and this North African treat fits the bill perfectly.

Serves 4

Contains 24 g of protein per serving

INGREDIENTS

4 tbsp olive oil
1 onion, finely diced
dash of salt
4 garlic cloves, crushed
2 red peppers, chopped
2 tsp sweet paprika
½ tsp cumin seeds
1 tsp cayenne pepper
2 x 400-g cans chopped tomatoes
4 eggs
1 handful of coriander leaves, chopped

METHOD

Place a large frying pan (that comes with a lid) over a medium heat, add the olive oil and gently sweat the onions with a pinch of salt. After 8-10 minutes, when soft and just golden, add the garlic, peppers and all the spices and fry until the peppers are starting to soften. Add the tomatoes, bring to the boil, then turn down the heat and simmer for 25-30 minutes.

With a spoon make four little dents in the sauce and break in the eggs. Season them with salt, turn the heat right down as low as possible, cover tightly with the lid and cook gently for 10 minutes until the egg yolks are just set. Sprinkle with coriander and serve.

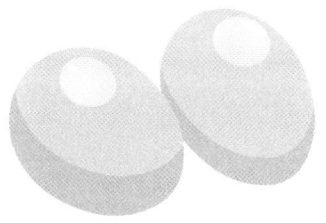

Buckwheat breakfast crêpe with eggs

Something for when you're trying to impress, perhaps, these buckwheat pancakes feel very French and have a touch of the long, relaxed holiday breakfast about them.

Serves 4

Contains 18 g of protein per serving

INGREDIENTS

100 g buckwheat flour
6 eggs
200 ml whole milk
1 tsp coconut oil
45 g Gruyère cheese, grated
pinch of salt

METHOD

Before you go to bed, simply combine the flour, 2 of the eggs and the milk and whisk to a smooth batter. Place in the fridge and leave until the morning.

Preheat the oven to 200°C and place a frying pan over a medium heat. To make the crêpes, melt a little coconut oil in the warm pan and wipe around with a kitchen towel so that only the thinnest film of oil is left in the pan. Spoon in a little pancake batter and tip the pan so that it covers the base of the pan. Cook for a minute on each side and then set aside while you make the rest of the crêpes. Next, on a lined baking sheet, simply lay out a pancake, place a small circle of Gruyère in the centre of the crêpe and crack an egg onto the cheese. Fold up the sides of the crêpe to create a little open-topped parcel and season with salt. Repeat for all four crêpes, then place in the hot oven for 5 minutes or until the yolks of the eggs are just set.

Apple, pecan and rye bircher muesli

Ideal for a quick breakfast, this can be prepped the night before, making it a perfect grab-and-go option in the morning.

Serves 2

Contains 9 g of protein per serving

INGREDIENTS

100 g rye oats
100 ml apple juice
2 apples, grated
100 ml whole milk
200 g strawberries, hulled and chopped
1 tbsp maple syrup
80 g Greek yoghurt
40 g pecans, chopped

METHOD

Start by mixing together the oats, apple juice, grated apple and milk. Cover and leave in the fridge for anywhere between 2 hours and overnight. Meanwhile, to make the compote, place a pan over a medium heat and toss in the chopped strawberries. Cook for 5 minutes until the strawberries are just breaking down, then remove from the heat and cool. When you are ready to eat, simply add the maple syrup to the soaked oats and serve with the yoghurt, pecans and strawberry compote.

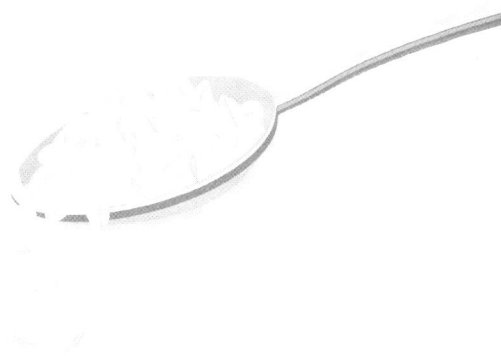

LUNCH

High-protein lunch recipes are where we can often have a bit of fun. Somehow there are fewer rules at lunchtime, meaning combining lots of proteins in one tasty dish is easy to achieve. In this chapter there are plenty of simple ideas to prep ahead of time or whip up on your lunch break. There are also some slightly more complex ideas that might work well for longer lunches, perhaps at the weekend or on leisurely days off. Be it a soup, salad or sandwich, this chapter has plenty of ideas for high-protein, high-flavour lunches to set you up perfectly for the rest of the day.

BLTA salad

We all know the magic of a BLT sandwich, so imagine removing the bread and adding avocado for all that joy but with more protein.

Serves 4

Contains 23 g of protein per serving

INGREDIENTS
FOR THE SALAD:

16 rashers pancetta or smoked streaky bacon

100 g baby spinach

2 little gem lettuces

400 g cherry tomatoes, halved

1 ripe avocado, sliced

FOR THE DRESSING:

1 large bunch of basil, leaves picked

100 g pine nuts

2 tbsp olive oil

1 lemon, juiced

1 garlic clove

METHOD

Preheat the oven to 200°C. Lay the pancetta in a single layer on a baking sheet and cook for 10 minutes until dark and crispy. While this cooks, blitz the basil, pine nuts, olive oil, lemon juice and garlic in a blender until they become a bright green paste. Place to one side and assemble the salad. Arrange the baby spinach and little gem lettuces on a platter and scatter over the cherry tomatoes. Remove the flesh from the avocado and slice it into the salad. Top this with spoonfuls of the basil dressing, and finally break the crispy pancetta over the salad.

Mussels with coconut, chilli and lime

A fresh, zingy treat to rustle up for a quick lunch, this mussel-heavy soup will put a spring in your step.

Serves 2

Contains 44 g of protein per serving

INGREDIENTS

1 kg mussels, cleaned
1 red chilli, chopped
1 x 400-ml can coconut milk
2 limes, juiced

METHOD

This dish could not be simpler. Place a heavy-bottomed saucepan over a high heat and get the pan nice and hot. Add the mussels to the hot pan and cover immediately with a lid. After 3 minutes, shake the pan vigorously, then lifting the lid, add the chilli and coconut milk and toss the mussels through the mix. Cook for a further minute or two, until all the mussels are open (discard any unopened mussels). Pour the lime juice over the top and serve immediately in large bowls.

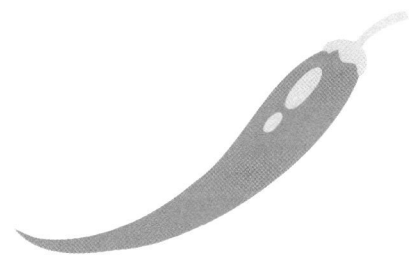

Salmon, broccoli, pomegranate and couscous salad

A crowd-pleaser if ever there was one. Combining three delicious sources of protein with couscous is always going to be a comforting high-protein winner.

Serves 2

Contains 37 g of protein per serving

INGREDIENTS

200 g Tenderstem broccoli

dash of salt

2 salmon fillets, skinned

100 g couscous

1 tbsp olive oil

2 tbsp pomegranate seeds

1 lemon, juiced

handful of mixed seeds

2 handfuls of watercress

METHOD

Bring a large pan of water to the boil, then add the broccoli and a good pinch of salt. Place a steamer basket or colander over the pan and place the salmon fillets into the steamer. Cover with a lid and cook the broccoli and salmon for 6 minutes. Remove the steamer basket and allow the salmon fillets to cool. Remove the broccoli from the water, but do not throw the water away. In a large bowl, add the couscous, a pinch of salt and the olive oil. Mix well and add enough of the broccoli cooking water to cover the couscous. Cover tightly and leave to steam for 10 minutes. When cooked, separate the couscous with a fork. To assemble the salad, combine the broccoli, pomegranate seeds, lemon juice, mixed seeds and watercress in a bowl and toss well. Turn out onto a platter or plates and top with the salmon fillets.

Salmon tacos

Reminiscent of tacos from a beachside shack in Baja California, but in the comfort of your own home, perhaps in your slippers, if you so wish.

Serves 2

Contains 32 g of protein per serving

INGREDIENTS

1 tbsp olive oil
2 tsp allspice
2 tsp paprika
¼ tsp sea salt
2 salmon fillets, skin on
1 handful of coriander leaves, chopped
1 handful of mint leaves, chopped
1 carrot, peeled into thin strips
6 radishes, finely sliced
½ fennel bulb, finely sliced
1 fresh red chilli, finely sliced
1 tbsp white wine vinegar
pinch of sugar
4 corn or flour tortillas

METHOD

Combine the oil, allspice, paprika and salt in a small bowl, then completely coat the salmon fillets with this mixture. Place a heavy-bottomed frying pan over a medium heat and put the salmon fillets skin-side down in the pan. Cook on the skin side for 6 minutes before turning onto the flesh side and cooking for a final 2 minutes. They will look slightly burnt, but don't panic; that is intentional! Next, in a mixing bowl, combine the coriander, mint, carrot, radishes, fennel and chilli. Add the vinegar and sugar and toss well to coat everything. To serve, place a tortilla on each plate and flake the salmon fillets, including any crispy skin, over the tortilla. Add a good handful of the crunchy salad and enjoy.

Smoked salmon, pickled cucumber and labneh on rye

A twist on a classic, swapping cream cheese for labneh, which helps boost our protein while also making this even more delicious.

Serves 2

Contains 24 g of protein per serving

INGREDIENTS

¼ tsp salt
250 g Greek yoghurt
150 ml white wine vinegar
150 ml water
75 g caster sugar
1 small cucumber, sliced
4 slices of rye bread
150 g smoked salmon

METHOD

Prepare the labneh one day in advance (it keeps for up to a week, so you could make a slightly larger batch). Mix the salt into the yoghurt and place into a tea towel, tie up the four corners of the towel and hang it from a tap over a sink overnight to draw out the moisture from the yoghurt to create a nice salty, fresh cheese. You can also purchase labneh in the supermarket or switch it for cream cheese here. To prepare the pickled cucumber, take a small heavy-bottomed saucepan and, over a medium heat, warm the vinegar, water and caster sugar until dissolved. Allow to cool before pouring this solution over the sliced cucumber. Leave for at least 1 hour to pickle. You can do this days in advance and it will last for up to a month in a sealed container in the fridge. When you are ready to eat, toast the rye bread before spreading a good amount of labneh on each slice. Top with smoked salmon and a few pickled cucumbers and enjoy.

Summer vegetable and goat's cheese frittata

This brings lovely fresh flavours to your table all year round. You could also consider using asparagus if desired.

Serves 2

Contains 26 g of protein per serving

INGREDIENTS

75 g French beans, roughly chopped
150 g frozen peas or small broad beans, shelled
6 eggs
pinch of salt
pinch of black pepper
3 sprigs mint, leaves picked and chopped
1 knob of unsalted butter
3 spring onions, sliced
40 g goat's cheese

METHOD

Preheat the oven to 180°C. Bring a pan of salted water to the boil and cook the beans for 4 minutes, adding the peas or broad beans for the final 2 minutes of cooking time. Drain all the veg in a colander and set aside. Whisk the eggs together with a pinch of salt and black pepper and most of the chopped mint. Melt the butter in an ovenproof frying pan, add the spring onions and cook gently for about 5 minutes until soft. Add the drained veg to the pan, then pour in the whisked eggs. Cook for 2 minutes before crumbling the goat's cheese over the top. Place in the oven for 6-8 minutes, until just set on top. Scatter the remaining mint on top and serve the frittata warm or cold with a green salad.

Grilled chicken with kale, pine nuts and Parmesan

Massaging the kale is key as it breaks down and softens the leaves while releasing more flavour. This has chicken Caesar salad vibes while delivering much more of a protein punch.

Serves 2

Contains 26 g of protein per serving

INGREDIENTS

2 skinless chicken breasts
1 tbsp olive oil, plus extra for grilling
1 bunch of kale
1 lemon, juiced
50 g Parmesan cheese, grated
dash of salt
dried chilli flakes
50 g pine nuts, toasted

METHOD

Preheat the grill to its highest setting. Place the chicken breasts on a foiled baking tray, coat them in a little olive oil and season on all sides with salt. Place under the grill for 5 minutes before turning and grilling on the other side for a further 5 minutes or until cooked through. While the chicken is grilling, wash and thoroughly dry the kale and remove the tough inner stems. Place the kale leaves in a large bowl and add 1 tbsp of olive oil, the lemon juice, half of the grated Parmesan and a good pinch of salt and dried chili flakes, as needed. Massage these ingredients into the kale quite roughly – you want the kale to start to break down, a little like if it were being cooked. After a minute or so of massage, the kale should be soft and more pliable. Slice the cooked chicken and serve with a pile of the massaged kale. Top with the rest of the Parmesan, the toasted pine nuts and another pinch of chilli flakes.

Tuna, avocado, ginger and lime poke

What's not to love about a poke bowl? Delicious, fresh, marinated fish tossed with vegetables and herbs, all hoovered up in a virtuous frenzy.

Serves 2

Contains 43 g of protein per serving

INGREDIENTS

250 g tuna steak, cut into 2-cm cubes
½ red onion, finely diced
2 cm ginger, peeled and grated
1 green chilli, finely diced
1 tbsp sesame oil
1 tbsp soya sauce
1 handful of coriander leaves, chopped
1 avocado, cut into 2-cm cubes
2 limes, juiced

METHOD

Combine all the ingredients in a bowl and leave to marinate for 30 minutes. Serve with some little gem lettuce to use as a scoop, or simply enjoy as it is.

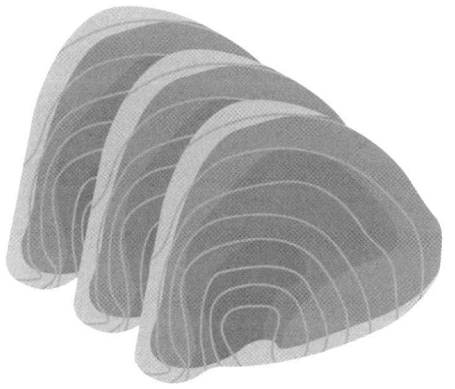

Roasted tofu with noodles

A dish this delicious should take more than 15 minutes to make from start to finish. This is quick and tasty, and includes ingredients that you likely have in your store cupboard already.

Serves 2

Contains 32 g of protein per serving

INGREDIENTS

250 g extra-firm tofu, cut into 2.5-cm cubes
2 tbsp soya sauce
1 tbsp sesame oil
1 cm ginger, grated
1 garlic clove, grated
150 g buckwheat soba noodles
1 red chilli, sliced
2 spring onions, sliced

METHOD

Preheat the oven to 200°C. In a large bowl, mix the tofu cubes, soya sauce, sesame oil, ginger and garlic, then tip onto a baking tray and cook in the hot oven for 10-12 minutes. Meanwhile, cook the noodles by soaking them in boiling water. When the tofu is cooked, simply toss it back into the mixing bowl, add the drained noodles and half of the sliced spring onion and chilli and mix. Divide between two plates and top with any leftover dressing and the rest of the spring onion and red chilli.

Gado gado

Gado gado is an Indonesian salad that brings together tasty, fresh ingredients and coats them in the most delicious peanut dressing you'll ever taste. That it's healthy and high in protein, too, elevates it to legendary status.

Serves 2

Contains 28 g of protein per serving

INGREDIENTS

400 g firm silken tofu
2 tbsp sesame oil
pinch of salt
400 g new potatoes, boiled and quartered
4 eggs, soft boiled and quartered
½ Chinese cabbage, shredded
2 ripe tomatoes, chopped
1 handful of radishes, roughly chopped, including leaves if you have them
½ cucumber, sliced
2 handfuls of bean sprouts
1 handful of coriander leaves, chopped
1 green chilli, sliced

FOR THE DRESSING:

1 garlic clove
50 g sugar
120 g crunchy peanut butter
2 red chillies
2 limes, juiced
¼ tsp salt
1 tbsp soya sauce
1 tbsp tamarind paste

METHOD

Cut the tofu into chunks, then warm the sesame oil in a frying pan over a medium heat. Fry the tofu in the sesame oil until golden, then sprinkle lightly with salt. For the dressing, put all the ingredients into a blender and blitz until smooth. Taste the seasoning, adding a little more lime or soya sauce as you see fit. To serve, simply layer the tofu, potatoes, eggs, cabbage, tomatoes, radishes, cucumber, bean sprouts, coriander and sliced chilli in a large bowl or on a platter and drizzle generously with the dressing.

DINNER

You have reached dinner time and want some high-protein meal ideas that are a step up from grilled chicken or salmon and rice or veggies. Luckily for you, in this chapter there are numerous interesting high-protein dinner recipes. Often at dinner time it is tempting to reach for the quick and easy carbohydrate-heavy option of pasta, pizza, or something speedy served with rice or potatoes. By borrowing from the cuisines of Italy, Greece, India and Thailand, this selection of recipes delivers big on protein, flavour and – most importantly – ease, meaning you'll be excited to get home to start cooking.

Lamb with tzatziki and chopped salad

Inspired by the flavours of Greece, this protein-packed dinner is a delicious treat to serve at the end of the day.

Serves 2

Contains 44 g of protein per serving

INGREDIENTS

4 lamb chops

FOR THE TZATZIKI:

½ cucumber, grated
½ garlic clove, grated
dash of salt
250 g Greek yoghurt

1 lemon, juiced
2 sprigs mint, leaves picked and chopped

FOR THE SALAD:

½ cucumber, chopped

2 large tomatoes, chopped

handful of black olives, pitted

50 g feta cheese, chopped

METHOD

Preheat the oven to 200°C. On a baking tray, season the lamb chops with a little olive oil and place in the hot oven for 15-20 minutes until cooked. While the lamb chops are cooking, make the tzatziki by placing the grated cucumber and garlic in a sieve with a little salt. After 5 minutes, squeeze as much liquid out of the cucumber as possible. Add this cucumber to the yoghurt and stir in a squeeze of lemon juice, a pinch of salt and the chopped mint. Set aside. For the salad, combine the cucumber, tomato and olives in a bowl. Season with the rest of the lemon juice, a little oil and a pinch of salt before topping with the chopped feta. Serve the lamb chops with some salad, a good spoonful of tzatziki and another liberal squeeze of lemon for good measure.

Baked Moroccan meatballs with couscous

Successfully combining supreme simplicity, big flavours and an impressive centrepiece for the table, these North African spiced meatballs are a winner for dinner.

Serves 4

Contains 30 g of protein per serving

INGREDIENTS

500 g beef mince
1 tsp ground cumin
1 tsp ground coriander
1 tsp dried chilli flakes
1 tsp salt
1 tsp black pepper
1 onion, peeled and sliced
2 garlic cloves, grated
250 g couscous
2 sprigs mint, leaves picked and chopped
75 g Greek yoghurt

METHOD

Preheat the oven to 200°C. In a mixing bowl, combine the beef mince, cumin, coriander, chilli flakes, salt and pepper. Shape tablespoonfuls of the mixture into meatballs. In a large ovenproof pan, fry the onion and garlic for 5 minutes before adding the meatballs and browning them all over. Next, add the couscous to the pan, along with enough water to just cover the meatballs. Place the pan, uncovered, in the oven and cook for 25-20 minutes until the couscous has absorbed all the water. Serve the baked meatballs and couscous with a nice sprinkling of chopped mint and a spoonful of yoghurt.

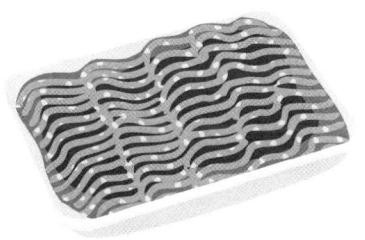

Moussaka

This recipe has a few stages, but it is worth it. This moussaka is protein-heavy and healthy, and is perfect for storing in the fridge and enjoying as a quick lunch, hot or cold, throughout the week.

Serves 4, with plenty of leftovers

Contains 31 g of protein per serving

INGREDIENTS

- 3 aubergines, cut lengthways into 1 cm-thick slices
- 2 tbsp olive oil
- pinch of salt
- 1 onion, sliced
- 2 garlic cloves, grated
- 1 tbsp dried oregano
- 1 lemon, zested
- 500 g lamb mince
- 100 g passata
- 300 ml low-fat crème fraîche
- 300 g Greek yoghurt
- 2 egg yolks
- 50 g Parmesan cheese

METHOD

Preheat the oven to 200°C. To start, lay the slices of aubergine on a baking tray and drizzle with 1 tbsp of olive oil and a good pinch of salt. Place in the oven for 20 minutes until starting to brown. Meanwhile, take a heavy-bottomed saucepan and place it over a medium heat. Add 1 tbsp of olive oil to the pan and, when hot, add the onions, garlic, dried oregano, lemon zest and a pinch of salt. Sweat for 5 minutes and then add the lamb mince. Brown this for a further 5 minutes before adding the passata and simmering for 20 minutes. Next, combine the crème fraîche, yoghurt, egg yolks and Parmesan in a bowl. In an ovenproof dish, start with a layer of aubergine, top with half of the lamb mince and finally half of the yoghurt mix. Repeat with the remaining ingredients, finishing with a layer of yoghurt mix. Bake for 40 minutes, or until the top is golden brown.

Cajun steak with coconut rice and beans

Perfectly spiced and with a richness from the coconut rice, this is one for when you want a high-protein meal that feels like a real treat.

Serves 2

Contains 54 g of protein per serving

INGREDIENTS

1 tsp paprika
1 tsp ground cumin
1 tsp ground coriander
1 tsp salt
1 tbsp olive oil
500 g rump steak, fat trimmed

100 g brown or red rice
200 g canned kidney beans
200 ml low-fat coconut milk
100 ml water

METHOD

Combine the paprika, cumin, coriander, salt and olive oil in a small bowl, then season the steak with this mixture. Leave to one side to marinate. Meanwhile, add the rice, kidney beans and their juice, along with the milk and 100 ml water, to a large pan and bring to the boil over a high heat. Once boiling, reduce to a simmer and cook for 30 minutes until the rice is soft to the bite and the liquid has all but disappeared. At this point, cover the pan with a lid and leave off the heat to steam. Place a frying pan over a high heat. When the pan starts to smoke, cook the steaks for 2 minutes per side and then let rest for 5 minutes out of the pan. Finally, slice the steaks and serve with the rice and beans and perhaps a little hot sauce if desired.

Thai beef salad

Cold noodles tossed with bright greens and a puckering dressing are the perfect foil for slivers of perfectly cooked steak.

Serves 4

Contains 30 g of protein per serving

INGREDIENTS

400 g vermicelli noodles

2 large rump steaks, fat trimmed

dash of salt

2 tsp sesame oil

½ cucumber, cut into batons

6 spring onions, sliced

2 little gem lettuces, quartered

1 large red chilli, sliced

FOR THE DRESSING:

1 tbsp soya sauce

1 tbsp rice wine vinegar

½ garlic clove, grated

1 cm ginger, grated

1 tsp dried chilli flakes

METHOD

Place the vermicelli in a bowl and cover with boiling water. Next, get a frying pan searingly hot, season the steak with salt and a little sesame oil on both sides, and cook on a high heat for 4 minutes on each side. Remove from the pan and allow to rest on a plate for at least 5 minutes. To make the dressing, combine the soya sauce, vinegar, garlic, ginger and dried chilli flakes. When you are ready to eat, simply drain the vermicelli and place into deep bowls. Top with a handful of each of the vegetables, a nice amount of sliced steak and a few slithers of sliced chilli, and dress with a generous slug of the dressing.

Paprika cod and steamed vegetables

This is a beautiful way to cook fish. It is so easy to prepare, and by cooking en papillote (in a pouch of baking paper) you lose nothing of the goodness in the fish nor the veg that steam beneath it.

Serves 2

Contains 19 g of protein per serving

INGREDIENTS

1 courgette, peeled into strips
1 red pepper, finely sliced
1 garlic clove, sliced
2 large tomatoes, chopped
2 cod fillets
2 tsp olive oil
pinch of salt
2 tsp paprika

METHOD

Preheat the oven to 200°C. Cut four 30 cm square sheets of baking parchment. Lay two sheets on top of each other, and place a pile of courgette, peppers, garlic and tomato in the centre of the parchment. Place the cod on top and season with salt and paprika. Bring together the top and bottom edges of the paper and fold over tightly to secure. Repeat with one of the edges. Add 1 tbsp water and fold over the final side to completely seal the parcel. Repeat with the other cod fillet and place both parcels on a baking sheet and then in the centre of the oven for 15 minutes. Remove from the oven and tear open the parcels. The fish should be perfectly cooked and the veg nicely steamed. Serve together and spoon a little of the sauce left in the bag over the top.

Lentil cassoulet

From four main ingredients and a bit of salt, oil and vinegar for seasoning, a classic is born. This is simpler than the French original, but it takes you most of the way there.

Serves 4

Contains 45 g of protein per serving

INGREDIENTS

2 x 400-g cans cooked green lentils
4 vine tomatoes, roughly chopped
1 tsp salt
1 tbsp red wine vinegar
8 sausages
4 skinless chicken thighs
2 tsp olive oil

METHOD

Preheat the oven to 200°C. In an ovenproof shallow saucepan, add the lentils and tomatoes and season with ½ tsp of salt and the vinegar. Bring to the boil, then turn down the heat and add the sausages and chicken thighs, seasoning the chicken with the remaining salt. Drizzle with the olive oil and place in the oven, uncovered, for 45 minutes. Remove when most of the liquid has evaporated and the chicken and sausages are golden brown. Serve on its own or with a green salad.

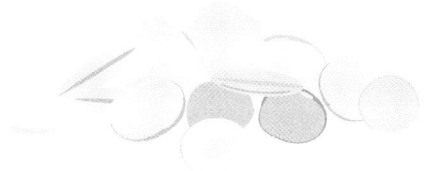

Tofu katsu curry

This is fun to make and delicious to eat, which stands it in pretty good stead for a dinner to make you smile.

Serves 2

Contains 25 g of protein per serving

INGREDIENTS

1 onion, diced
3 garlic cloves, grated
2 carrots, grated
2 tbsp plain flour
1 tbsp curry powder
1 tbsp garam masala
1 tbsp soya sauce
3 tbsp agave syrup
50 g cornflour
3 tbsp sesame oil
100 g panko breadcrumbs
400 g firm tofu, sliced into 1 cm-thick pieces
600 ml water
200 g cooked brown rice

METHOD

Add the onion, garlic and carrots to a saucepan over a medium heat. Add a tablespoon of water and cook, stirring occasionally, for 6-8 minutes. Add the flour, curry powder, garam masala, soya sauce and 2 tbsp of the agave syrup and cook for a further 6-8 minutes. While the sauce is cooking, find three shallow bowls. Add the cornflour to the first bowl; 1 tbsp sesame oil and 1 tbsp agave syrup to the second bowl; and the breadcrumbs to the final bowl. Next, place each slice of tofu in the cornflour, then the sesame oil and then the breadcrumbs, making sure each slice is well coated each time.

Next, add the 600 ml water to the sauce and leave to simmer for 10-15 minutes while you cook the tofu. Warm the two remaining tablespoons of sesame oil in a frying pan over a medium heat and fry the breaded tofu for 2 minutes on each side until golden brown. To serve, add some brown rice to each plate, top with a couple of bits of tofu and plenty of the delicious curry sauce.

Chilli paneer curry

A curry house classic, this couldn't be simpler to make at home. It packs a pleasing punch, and it is rich in protein from the paneer.

Serves 4

Contains 20 g of protein per serving

INGREDIENTS

1 tbsp olive oil
400 g firm paneer
2 tsp cumin seeds
2 garlic cloves, grated
2 green chillies, finely sliced
4 spring onions, finely sliced
dash of salt
1 lemon, juiced
1 x 400-g can coconut milk
1 handful of coriander leaves, chopped
4 wholemeal chapatis

METHOD

Warm a large frying pan over a high heat and add the olive oil. When hot, fry the paneer until golden brown on all sides. Add the cumin, garlic, green chillies and half the spring onions to the pan with a good pinch of salt and 2 tbsp of water. Toss together and cook until the water has all but evaporated. Finally, add the lemon juice and coconut milk and bring to the boil. Lower the heat and simmer for 15-20 minutes until you have a nice thick sauce that coats the paneer. Just before you are ready to eat, warm the chapatis. To serve, sprinkle the rest of the spring onions and the chopped coriander over the curry and eat with the chapatis.

Peruvian beef brisket broth, sweetcorn and cabbage

From the list of ingredients you might imagine this to be slightly dull, but the alchemy that comes from a long, slow cook makes this a very moreish high-protein dinner.

Serves 4

Contains 84 g of protein per serving

INGREDIENTS

600 g rolled beef brisket
pinch of salt
black pepper
2 onions, cut into wedges
2 bay leaves
2 cobs of sweetcorn, cut into 5-cm pieces
1 sweetheart cabbage, cut into wedges
½ tsp dried oregano

METHOD

Season the brisket all over with salt and pepper and place in a large saucepan that comes with a lid. Cover with cold water and place over a medium heat. Add the onions and bay leaves and bring to the boil. Immediately turn down the heat, cover and simmer for 1 hour and 30 minutes. Once cooked, add the sweetcorn and sweetheart cabbage to the pot and continue to simmer for a further 20 minutes. Add the dried oregano and some more salt and pepper if needed. To serve, add some cabbage and sweetcorn to each person's bowl and fill with broth. Slice the brisket and serve three or four slices per portion.

Pearl barley paella with chicken and prawns

Anyone familiar with Spanish cuisine will know the pulling power of a good paella. Imagine all of that here, with a pearl barley protein boost instead of the usual rice.

Serves 4

Contains 44 g of protein per serving

INGREDIENTS

1 tbsp olive oil

500 g chicken thigh fillets, roughly chopped

dash of salt

black pepper

1 red onion, finely chopped

2 long red chillies, deseeded and finely chopped

2 garlic cloves, crushed

1 tbsp sweet paprika

300 g pearl barley

375 ml water

12 frozen king prawns

1 lemon, quartered

METHOD

Heat the olive oil in a large frying pan over high heat. Add the chicken thighs to the pan, season each piece with salt and pepper, and brown all over until golden. Transfer to a bowl. In the same pan, add a little more oil if needed and the onion, chopped chillies, garlic and paprika, with a generous pinch of salt, and sweat for 8-10 minutes until translucent. Add the pearl barley and stir to combine before placing the chicken thighs and prawns into the pan. Pour over the water and bring to the boil. Turn down to a gentle simmer, cover with foil and cook for 30 minutes, or until the liquid is absorbed and the pearl barley is tender. Remove from the heat and set aside for 5 minutes to rest. Serve with a good squeeze of lemon.

Blackened broccoli with steamed fish and tahini sauce

The intense smoky sweetness of burning broccoli is the perfect contrast to simple steamed fish and the richness of tahini.

Serves 2

Contains 25 g of protein per serving

INGREDIENTS

1 head broccoli
2 tbsp olive oil
2 tsp dried chilli flakes
pinch of salt
¼ garlic clove
2 tbsp tahini
2 lemons, juiced
2 white fish fillets (sea bass, sea bream, haddock or cod would work well)

METHOD

Preheat the oven to 200°C. Cut the head of broccoli into eight long spears. Toss these with 1 tbsp of olive oil, 1 tsp of chilli flakes and ¼ tsp salt, and spread out on a roasting tray. Place in the top of the preheated oven and cook for 30-40 minutes, turning halfway through, until starting to blacken. While the broccoli is roasting, take a pestle and mortar (or a blender) and crush the garlic with a pinch of salt. Add the tahini and mix before adding the lemon juice. The paste will thicken as you mix in the lemon juice. Slowly add the remaining 1 tbsp of oil, mixing all the time, before adding 1-2 tbsp warm water to loosen the sauce to the consistency of single cream.

Finally, season the fillets of fish with salt and steam for 8-10 minutes (depending on the thickness of the fish), until just cooked through. To serve, arrange the broccoli and steamed fish on a plate and drizzle liberally with the tahini sauce.

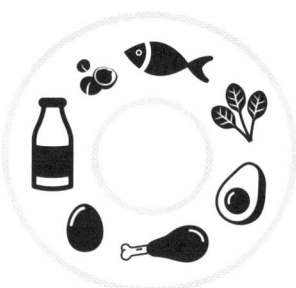

DESSERT

Desserts? Surely not. Au contraire – of course there are desserts. Following any diet should never limit the joy you can have with cooking and eating. In fact, by finishing a meal with an exciting protein-packed treat, you'll be ensuring you're fully sated, and with good, satisfying proteins to keep you fuller for longer. You don't have to miss out on things you'd assume might be off the menu. We've got ice creams, chocolate mousse, tiramisu and more to help you finish off a meal with a bang. Of course, not all meals need the fireworks of a big fancy dessert. Yoghurt and fruit, for instance, are a great way to round off a meal and deliver a protein top-up at the same time.

Mango and chia seed ice cream

This delicious ice cream is free of added sugars, protein packed and vegan, which makes it a unicorn in the dessert world.

Serves 4

Contains 17 g of protein per serving

INGREDIENTS

2 scoops whey protein powder
240 ml almond milk
6 tbsp chia seeds
2 ripe mangoes, peeled and cut into chunks

METHOD

Mix together the protein powder, almond milk and chia seeds, and leave in the refrigerator for at least 30 minutes. Once the chia seeds have absorbed some of the almond milk and the mix is a little firm, tip this into a blender or food processor with three-quarters of the chopped mango and blitz to a smooth paste. Pour the mix into a shallow tray or Tupperware, cover and place in the freezer for at least 4 hours, removing every hour or so and stirring with a fork to ensure a smooth ice cream with not too many large ice crystals. Once frozen completely, scoop into individual bowls and top with the remaining chunks of mango.

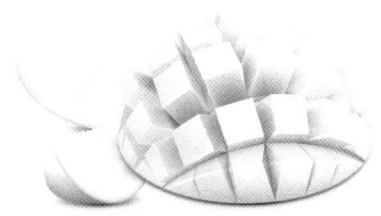

Coconut and pineapple frozen yoghurt

This frozen yoghurt is so rich and zingy you'll be making double batches and visiting the freezer in the middle of the night before you know what has happened to you.

Serves 4

Contains 13 g of protein per serving

INGREDIENTS

500 g Greek yoghurt
50 g coconut sugar
50 g desiccated coconut
2 lemons, zested and juiced
1 pineapple, peeled and chopped

METHOD

Combine all the ingredients in a blender or food processor and blitz until the mixture is smooth. Pour into a shallow tray or Tupperware, cover and pop in the freezer for at least 4 hours, removing every hour or so and stirring with a fork to ensure a smooth finished result with not too many large ice crystals. Once frozen completely, scoop into individual bowls and top with some extra desiccated coconut and lemon zest if you fancy.

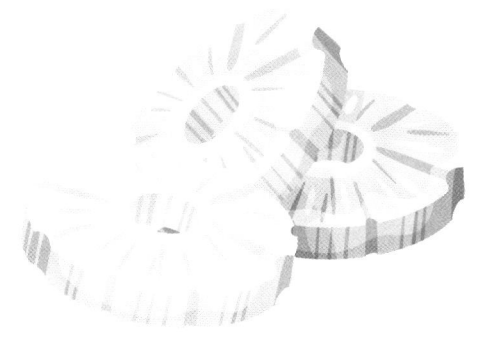

Tiramisu

By switching out some of the mascarpone, sugar and biscuits, and bringing chia, yoghurt and rice cakes to the party instead, you get a delicious dessert that brings protein to the table in bucketloads.

Serves 4

Contains 35 g of protein per serving

INGREDIENTS

4 tbsp chia seeds
2 tbsp Greek yoghurt
300 ml milk
200 ml black coffee
4 tbsp cocoa powder
1 tsp vanilla extract
8 chocolate-covered rice cakes

METHOD

Place the chia seeds, yoghurt and milk in a lidded jar or container and shake vigorously. Put to one side. Make the coffee and pour into a shallow bowl or baking tray along with 3 tbsp of cocoa powder and the vanilla extract and mix until smooth. Soak the rice cakes in the liquid for a moment and then drain them onto a plate. In a serving dish, create a layer of the creamy chia seeds, top with the soaked rice cakes, and repeat until you have used up all of the mixture, making sure the top layer is the creamy chia seed mixture. Dust the whole thing with the remaining cocoa powder and chill in the fridge overnight (or for at least 1 hour).

Chocolate mousse

Who doesn't love chocolate mousse? This one delivers on protein as well as flavour and is as light as falling snow. It will leave you howling for more.

Serves 4

Contains 10 g of protein per serving

INGREDIENTS

300 ml double cream
3 tbsp cocoa powder
2 scoops protein powder
2 tbsp agave syrup
½ tsp vanilla extract
25 g dark chocolate, grated

METHOD

Place all the ingredients except the dark chocolate in a large mixing bowl and whisk with a hand whisk until light and fluffy. Portion into little pots and refrigerate for 30 minutes. Grate the dark chocolate over the top and enjoy.

Baked ricotta and figs

A very grown-up dessert, this is reminiscent of an autumnal evening in Tuscany and is a nice treat after a hearty meal.

Serves 2

Contains 13 g of protein per serving

INGREDIENTS

250 g round of ricotta
1 tsp caster sugar
4 figs, halved
2 tbsp honey

METHOD

Preheat the oven to 200°C. Simply turn out the ricotta from its container onto a lined baking tray and top with the caster sugar. Place the figs around the ricotta and drizzle with the honey. Bake in the hot oven for 25 minutes until the ricotta is firm and golden brown and the figs have collapsed and turned jammy. Divide between two bowls and enjoy.

Sweet potato and pecan pudding

For something so rich and seemingly decadent, this pudding is surprisingly good for you and has an unexpectedly healthy amount of protein to boot.

Serves 4

Contains 7 g of protein per serving

INGREDIENTS

100 g unsalted butter

200 g baked sweet potato, flesh scooped out

2 tbsp maple syrup

1 tbsp raw cacao nibs

2 tbsp cocoa powder

2 eggs

2 tsp vanilla extract

100 g ground almonds

¼ tsp baking powder

100 g chopped pecans

½ tsp salt

2 tbsp whey protein powder

METHOD

Line an 18 cm baking tin with parchment or foil and preheat the oven to 160°C. First, melt the butter in a small saucepan. Next, beat the sweet potato flesh with the maple syrup until smooth, then mix in the melted butter, cacao nibs and cocoa powder. Add the eggs and vanilla extract, beat until thick, then stir in the ground almonds, baking powder, pecans, salt and whey protein. Spoon into the lined baking tin and bake for about 20-25 minutes, until just cooked and still soft under the crust. Serve while still warm, perhaps with a spoonful of yoghurt if you fancy.

SNACKS

Eating a high-protein diet should mean you stay fuller for longer and don't have so many mid-morning or mid-afternoon cravings. However, it is important to have a few go-to nibbles up your sleeve so that a good protein-rich snack is always within reach when the inevitable snack craving does descend. You can, of course, have a few saviours in your store cupboard, such as jerky; fruit, nut and seed trail mix; hard-boiled eggs or even protein bars and balls. But equally, having a reliable arsenal of high-protein shakes, cakes, snacks and cookies to call on is only a good thing, and they should fill that hole that often only a sugary cookie or brownie can fill.

Chocolate and peanut butter shake

Whether to satisfy a post-workout or between-meal hunger, this delicious, protein-packed shake will stop you from reaching for a chocolate bar or biscuit when the craving strikes.

Serves 1

Contains 49 g of protein per serving

INGREDIENTS

2 scoops chocolate-flavoured protein powder
140 ml whole milk

1 banana
2 tbsp peanut butter
3 ice cubes

METHOD

Add everything to a blender and blitz until smooth.

Peanut and coconut flapjacks

These are not only protein packed, but also very simple to make and require no cooking – an absolute godsend.

Serves 12

Contains 11 g of protein per serving

INGREDIENTS

2 scoops protein powder
170 g peanut butter
250 ml agave syrup
100 g rolled oats
200 g coconut flour

METHOD

Add all the ingredients to a bowl and mix. Line a baking tray and press the mixture into it in a solid flat layer. Refrigerate for at least 40 minutes. Cut into squares and eat immediately or store in Tupperware in the fridge and eat as and when you need an energy boost.

Double chocolate and macadamia nut cookies

These are undoubtedly chocolate cookies and should be treated as such, so don't go overboard. However, as far as cookies go, they don't get much better for you than this.

Serves 8

Contains 10 g of protein per serving

INGREDIENTS

- 120 g brown rice flour
- 2 scoops protein powder
- 25 g coconut sugar
- 1 tsp baking powder
- 1 tbsp coconut oil
- 30 g Greek yoghurt
- 1 egg, beaten
- 1 tbsp cacao powder
- 25 g white chocolate chips
- 25 g macadamia nuts, chopped

METHOD

Preheat the oven to 180°C. Mix all the ingredients together to form a nice firm dough. Roll spoonfuls of the dough into balls and place on a baking tray lined with baking parchment. Bake in the hot oven for 15 minutes. Allow to cool before tucking in.

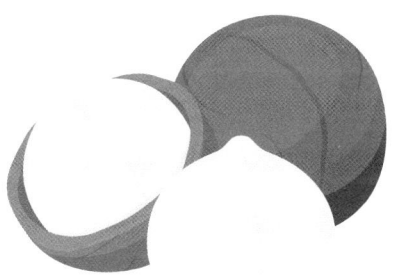

Tahini and lime roasted kale chips

Sometimes you just want to rip open a bag of crisps and dig in. Well, now you can. These perfectly crisped kale leaves are as zingy and delicious as any potato crisp out there.

Serves 4

Contains 5 g of protein per serving

INGREDIENTS

1 large bunch of kale
2 tbsp lime juice
4 tbsp tahini
2 tbsp olive oil
1 tsp dried chilli flakes
½ tsp salt

METHOD

Preheat the oven to 100°C and line a baking tray with foil or parchment. Wash and thoroughly dry the kale, then remove the tough inner stems. Tear the leaves into roughly 3 cm pieces and place in a large bowl. In a small bowl, whisk together the lime juice, tahini, oil, dried chilli and salt. Pour this over the kale and massage the marinade into the leaves. Spread the leaves in a single layer on the baking tray and place in the oven. Start to check on them after 30 minutes, although they could take up to an hour to become crispy. They are ready when the seasonings are completely dry and the kale is crispy.

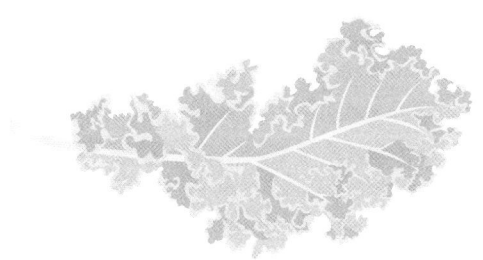

Salmon and cucumber hand rolls

Smaller pieces of these fresh, protein-packed rolls work perfectly for a snack, or you could leave it whole and eat it like a wrap for a more substantial lunch.

Serves 8

Contains 16 g of protein per serving

INGREDIENTS

180 g sushi rice
350 ml water
60 ml rice wine vinegar
2 tsp vegetable oil
25 g caster sugar
1 tsp salt
1 sheet nori seaweed
½ cucumber, cut into thin batons
1 salmon fillet, skinned and thinly sliced

METHOD

Wash the rice until the water runs clear. Transfer into a medium saucepan and cover with 350 ml of water. Bring to the boil, reduce the heat to low, cover with a lid and cook for 20 minutes. Meanwhile, combine the rice wine vinegar, oil, sugar and salt in a small pan and warm until the sugar dissolves. Pour the rice onto a flat baking tray to allow it to cool quickly, then pour the vinegar mixture on top and work into the rice with your hands. Place the seaweed on a board, rough side up, and take a handful of rice and spread it on the seaweed along the edge nearest to you. Place the cucumber and salmon across the middle of the rice and roll up the seaweed lengthways. Cut into sections and eat immediately, or refrigerate and eat as a snack or part of a healthy lunch.

No-cook pistachio, cardamom and cranberry granola bars

Another one for the no-cook snack gang, these are packed with fruits, nuts and spices, and are completely moreish, so make a batch and tuck in.

Serves 12

Contains 10 g of protein per serving

INGREDIENTS

200 g dates, pitted
135 g rolled oats
110 g pistachios, roughly chopped
75 g mixed seeds
75 g dried cranberries

2 tbsp protein powder
1 tsp ground cardamom
100 g honey
100 g smooth peanut butter

METHOD

Chop the dates as small as you can, then add to a large mixing bowl along with the oats, pistachios, seeds, cranberries, protein powder and cardamom. Warm the honey and peanut butter in a small saucepan over a low heat. Stir, then pour over the oat mixture and mix, breaking up the dates to disperse throughout. Once thoroughly mixed, transfer to a 20 cm baking dish or other small pan lined with cling film or parchment. Press the mixture down firmly until uniformly flattened, cover with cling film and let it firm up in the fridge or freezer for 15-20 minutes. Once firm, chop into 10-12 even bars. These will last stored in an airtight container for a few days.

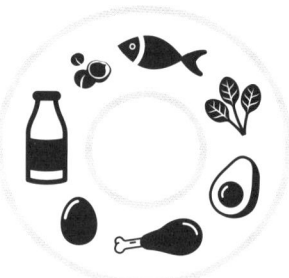

MEAL PLANNERS

In this chapter, you'll find a three-week meal planner to help you get started on your protein journey. Feel free to substitute other protein-friendly ingredients and mix and match meals from different days. Most importantly, create a plan you will enjoy and stick to and one that will help you reap the rewards of this diet!

MEAL PLANNER – WEEK ONE

	MONDAY	**TUESDAY**	**WEDNESDAY**
BREAKFAST	Toasted breakfast bread (p.32) with cottage cheese and mango	Pear and walnut oats with pumpkin seeds	Very berry breakfast bowl (p.35)
LUNCH	Tuna, cucumber, feta and bulghur wheat salad	Hummus, falafel and spinach wrap	Smoked salmon, pickled cucumber and labneh on rye (p.52)
DINNER	Pearl barley paella with chicken and prawns (p.86)	Baked sweet potato with tuna and cottage cheese	Thai beef salad (p.74)
DESSERT/ SNACKS	Peanut and coconut flapjacks (p.105)	Salmon and cucumber hand rolls (p.110)	No-cook pistachio, cardamom and cranberry granola bars (p.112)

THURSDAY	FRIDAY	SATURDAY	SUNDAY
Greek yoghurt with chopped nuts and compote	Apple, pecan and rye bircher muesli (p.40)	Scrambled eggs with smoked salmon and rye bread	Mexican divorced eggs (p.30)
Chicken enchiladas	BLTA salad (p.44)	Summer vegetable and goat's cheese frittata (p.54)	Grilled chicken with kale, pine nuts and Parmesan (p.56)
Moussaka (p.70)	Tofu katsu curry (p.80)	Lamb with tzatziki and chopped salad (p.66)	Roasted veg, couscous, walnuts and Halloumi
Tahini and lime roasted kale chips (p.108)	Date and pistachio protein balls	Coconut and pineapple frozen yoghurt (p.94)	Sweet potato and pecan pudding (p.100)

MEAL PLANNER – WEEK TWO

	MONDAY	TUESDAY	WEDNESDAY
BREAKFAST	Toasted breakfast bread (p.32) with almond butter, sliced banana and pumpkin seeds	Greek yoghurt, walnuts, honey and berries	Mexican chia and chocolate breakfast shake (p.34)
LUNCH	Salmon tacos (p.50)	Chopped chicken, freekeh, pomegranate and tahini salad	Roasted tofu with noodles (p.60)
DINNER	Steamed chicken, almond and brown rice pilaf, tahini sauce	Chilli paneer curry (p.82)	Baked sweet potato with cowboy beans (p.28) and grated cheddar
DESSERT/ SNACKS	Tahini and lime roasted kale chips (p.108)	Salmon and cucumber hand rolls (p.110)	Date and pistachio protein balls

THURSDAY	FRIDAY	SATURDAY	SUNDAY
Rye bread, ricotta scrambled eggs and avocado	Apple and cinnamon oats with chopped pecans	Cowboy beans and poached eggs (p.28)	Buckwheat breakfast crêpe with eggs (p.38)
Chili paneer, cucumber raita and fresh mango wrap	Tuna, avocado, ginger and lime poke (p.58)	Chicken Caesar salad with rye bread croutons and anchovies	Poached salmon with roasted beetroot, feta and walnuts
Blackened broccoli with steamed fish and tahini sauce (p.88)	Baked Moroccan meatballs and couscous (p.68)	Paprika cod and steamed vegetables (p.76)	Lamb chops, hummus and tabbouleh
Mango chia pudding	Peanut and coconut flapjacks (p.105)	Baked ricotta and figs (p.99)	Tiramisu (p.96)

MEAL PLANNER – WEEK THREE

	MONDAY	**TUESDAY**	**WEDNESDAY**
BREAKFAST	Toasted breakfast bread (p.32) with ricotta, honey and figs	Mexican chia and chocolate breakfast shake (p.34)	Bircher muesli with strawberry compote (p.40)
LUNCH	BLTA salad (p.44)	Smoked salmon, pickled cucumber and labneh on rye (p.52)	Salmon, broccoli, pomegranate and couscous salad (p.48)
DINNER	Moussaka (p.70)	Roasted sweet potato with chilli con carne	Chicken katsu curry
DESSERT/ SNACKS	Peanut and coconut flapjacks (p.105)	Tahini and lime roasted kale chips (p.108)	Double chocolate and macadamia nut cookies (p.106)

THURSDAY	FRIDAY	SATURDAY	SUNDAY
Greek yoghurt with banana, cacao and coconut flakes	Dark chocolate, blackberry and chia overnight oats	Shakshuka and baked eggs (p.36)	Scrambled eggs with smoked salmon and rye bread
Smoked turkey, tomato and mozzarella wholewheat wrap	Asparagus and goat's cheese frittata	Gado gado (p.62)	Mussels with coconut, chilli and lime (p.46)
Baked Moroccan meatballs and couscous (p.68)	Lentil cassoulet (p.78)	Cajun steak with coconut rice and beans (p.72)	Peruvian beef brisket broth, sweetcorn and cabbage (p.84)
Kiwi, spinach and chia shake	Salmon and cucumber hand rolls (p.110)	Mango and chia seed ice cream (p.92)	Chocolate mousse (p.98)

CONCLUSION

Hopefully now you've learned the basics and some staple protein recipes, you'll feel confident switching to a high-protein diet.

Many high-protein-diet disciples espouse prosaic recipes that struggle to inspire all but the hardiest high-protein aficionados to eat in this way. However, there is a broad spectrum of foods that contain plenty of protein, and bringing them together in delicious and inventive ways means you can have a high-protein diet that excites, entices and also nourishes you and those around you.

It is important to remember two things. Firstly, eating as broad of a diet as possible is always going to be more delicious and better for you. So don't just get all your protein from one source – mix it up, try new things. Secondly, non-processed whole foods are your friend – unsweetened yoghurt, milk, eggs, nuts, seeds and plenty of beans, pulses, fruit and veg will always stand you in good stead, be it in your pursuit of a high-protein diet or simply in your pursuit of eating better. May your journey towards eating a high-protein-diet be both delicious and nutritious!

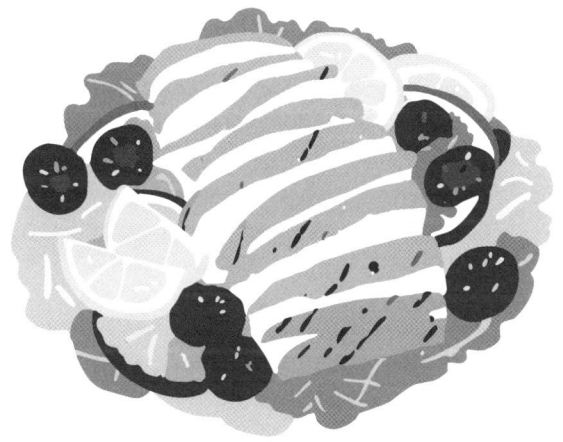

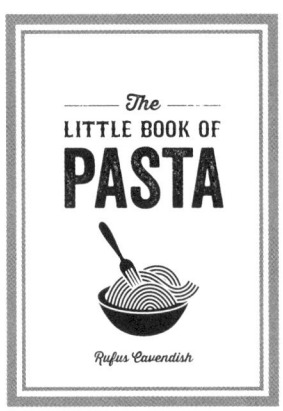

The Little Book of Pasta
A Pocket Guide to Italy's Favourite Food, Featuring History, Trivia, Recipes and More

Rufus Cavendish

Paperback • ISBN: 978-1-80007-841-3

Whether fresh, dried, baked into lasagna or swirled as spaghetti around your fork, pasta is fantastic. From farfalle and fusilli to fettucine and beyond, this pocket guide serves up a celebration of one of the world's most popular foods. With history, trivia, tips and recipes, it's got all the information and inspiration you could hunger for.

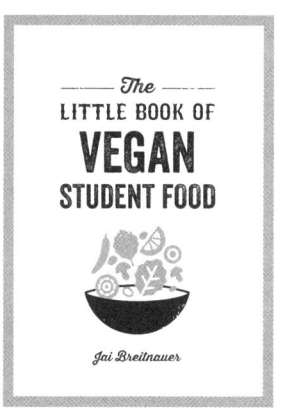

The Little Book of Vegan Student Food
Easy Vegan Recipes for Tasty, Healthy Eating on a Budget

Jai Breitnauer

Paperback • ISBN: 978-1-83799-276-8

A pocket-sized guide to all things vegan grub, this little book is the perfect gift for students. Featuring an array of budget-friendly, flavourful and easy-to-make meals, this book gives you the vegan recipes you need to spice up your student suppers.

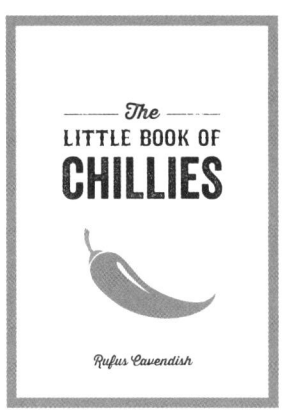

The Little Book of Chillies
A Pocket Guide to the Wonderful World of Chilli Peppers, Featuring Recipes, Trivia and More

Rufus Cavendish

Paperback • ISBN: 978-1-80007-416-3

This book is a celebration of the all-conquering capsicum – from mild varieties to red-hot peppers – served with a spicy side of trivia, tips and recipes. The perfect pocket guide to these wonders of nature, it explores how they became so widely loved, where their heat comes from, and how they can beguile and benefit our bodies.

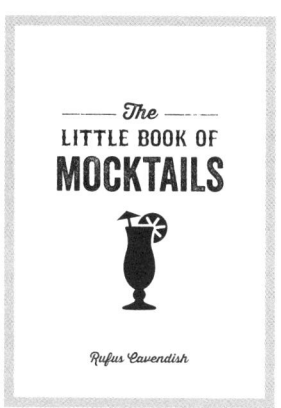

The Little Book of Mocktails
Delicious Alcohol-Free Recipes for Any Occasion

Rufus Cavendish

Paperback • ISBN: 978-1-80007-150-6

Master the art of the mocktail with this classy concoction of recipes and tips for deliciously booze-free beverages. Whether you're ditching alcohol completely or just looking for healthier alternatives, let these teetotal tipples dazzle and delight your taste buds!

Have you enjoyed this book? If so, find us on Facebook at **SUMMERSDALE PUBLISHERS**, on Twitter/X at **@SUMMERSDALE** and on Instagram and TikTok at **@SUMMERSDALEBOOKS** and get in touch. We'd love to hear from you!

WWW.SUMMERSDALE.COM

IMAGE CREDITS

Cover images: avocado, milk, spinach, egg © RedKoala/Shutterstock.com; fish © Pixelz Studio/Shutterstock.com; chicken © Aleksandr_Lysenko/Shutterstock.com

p.33 © aiselmisha/Shutterstock.com

p.37 aiselmisha/Shutterstock.com

p.41 © Johnny Dream/Shutterstock.com

p.47 © serazetdinov/Shutterstock.com

p.59 © Kidung Paripurna/Shutterstock.com

p.61 © judyjump/Shutterstock.com

p.69 © Luis Line/Shutterstock.com

p.75 © Sunnydream/Shutterstock.com

p.79 © Toltemara/Shutterstock.com

p.85 © Vector Tradition/Shutterstock.com

p.93 © albe_ga/Shutterstock.com

p.95 © HappyPictures/Shutterstock.com

p.107 © Rinat Sultanov/Shutterstock.com

p.109 © Sunnydream/Shutterstock.com

p.123 © S chana/Shutterstock.com